Distribution, publication, and copying in any form are prohibited and subject to damages.

TEN HYPNOSES

Copying, publishing, and sharing with third parties are only permitted with the written consent of the author. Please observe the notes on copyright and usage.

Distribution, publication, and copying in any form are prohibited and subject to damages.

Copying, publishing, and sharing with third parties are only permitted with the written consent of the author. Please observe the notes on copyright and usage.

Distribution, publication, and copying in any form are prohibited and subject to damages.

Ingo Michael Simon

TEN HYPNOSES

11

Psychosomatics

Copying, publishing, and sharing with third parties are only permitted with the written consent of the author. Please observe the notes on copyright and usage.

Distribution, publication, and copying in any form are prohibited and subject to damages.

© 2024 Ingo Michael Simon
All rights reserved.
Independently published
www.ingosimon.com

Important Notes for Urgent Attention:
The contents of this book are based on the practical experiences of the author with hypnosis applications and psychotherapy in a trance state. Although the author has strived for the utmost care, errors or misunderstandings in the presentation cannot be completely excluded. Therapeutic work with people and the application of hypnosis are solely the responsibility of the hypnotist. It cannot be ruled out that parts of this book may be misunderstood or that the application of a presented procedure may cause an undesirable reaction in the client. The author also assumes no co-responsibility if work with a client is carried out with reference to the statements in this book.

The Author:
Ingo Michael Simon studied psychology and education and is a hypnotherapist with practices in southwestern Germany and Switzerland. With the help of hypnosis-supported psychotherapy, he primarily treats people with persistent psychological conditions. His practice focuses on anxiety disorders, pathological compulsions, and psychosomatic illnesses. His therapeutic offerings mainly include classical and modern hypnosis applications and the dreamland therapy he developed himself.

Copying, publishing, and sharing with third parties are only permitted with the written consent of the author. Please observe the notes on copyright and usage.

Distribution, publication, and copying in any form are prohibited and subject to damages.

Notes on Copyright and Usage

Copying, publishing, and sharing with third parties is prohibited and only permitted with the written consent of the author. Please observe the following copyright and usage guidelines.

This work has been carefully crafted and created to the best of the author's knowledge and personal experience. It comprises text templates and application guidelines for professional hypnosis sessions. The author is a licensed psychotherapist with extensive experience in psychotherapy, coaching, and personal training using hypnotic techniques and methods. Nevertheless, the author and the publisher assume no liability for the accuracy of information, instructions, and advice, nor for any typographical errors. The author and publisher accept no responsibility or liability for the application of these texts and recommendations with clients or patients, nor for any potential consequences or unexpected reactions. It is expressly noted that the application of therapeutic and advisory techniques and formulations lies solely and entirely within the responsibility of the practitioner. This also applies to adherence to the boundaries of legally regulated medical and therapeutic practices. The fact that a book containing action proposals is freely available for sale does not imply that its application with clients or patients is permitted for everyone.

Distribution, publication, and copying in any form are prohibited and subject to damages.

Copying, publishing, and sharing with third parties are only permitted with the written consent of the author. Please observe the notes on copyright and usage.

Distribution, publication, and copying in any form are prohibited and subject to damages.

Table of Contents

Introduction 9

#1 11

#2 16

#3 21

#4 27

#5 33

#6 38

#7 43

#8 48

#9 52

#10 57

Overview of All Titles in the Series "Ten Hypnoses" 62

Copying, publishing, and sharing with third parties are only permitted with the written consent of the author. Please observe the notes on copyright and usage.

Distribution, publication, and copying in any form are prohibited and subject to damages.

Copying, publishing, and sharing with third parties are only permitted with the written consent of the author. Please observe the notes on copyright and usage.

Introduction

The series "Ten Hypnoses" is very well known in Germany, Austria, and Switzerland as a collection of texts for therapeutic work and is used by numerous psychotherapeutic practices, doctors, therapists, coaches, and other helping professionals. I am pleased to now be able to offer these texts in other countries as well.

Most therapists have their own methods for inducing and deepening trance as well as for exiting trance. Therefore, I have focused on the main part of the hypnosis. The texts in this book can be integrated as the main part into any hypnosis process.

The texts in this collection use various hypnosis techniques. I will not explain these in detail, as I assume that users have the appropriate training. It is also not necessary to understand the exact structure or functioning of the different parts. The texts can simply be read aloud, and they will have their effect.

Decide for yourself which text best suits your client or patient at any given time. You can also combine passages from different texts. It is not about using all ten hypnoses in sequence. It is a selection of possibilities.

I want to emphasize that books cannot replace therapy. Psychotherapy or other therapeutic treatments involve much more. A careful diagnosis is the necessary basis for deciding on the use of methods, including whether hypnosis or one of my texts should be used. Even in this case, preparatory discussions, follow-up discussions during the session, and of course, a therapeutic concept for the sequence of sessions and the content approaches are essential parts of therapy. This cannot and should not be achieved with a collection of texts.

In any case, I wish you much success in your work and I am pleased if my text templates can contribute in a small way.

Ingo Michael Simon

#1

You have dealt with your illness and you know that it now depends to adjust yourself to getting well again ... ... to align your inner being with it, as best as you can, to let go of the illness and all the backgrounds and causes that exist... ... to fully adjust to healing again ... ... as best as possible ... ... as far as possible ... ... Most of the time, even with difficult illnesses, there is much more improvement, relief and also healing is more possible than we think ... ... and you have decided to achieve everything that is possible ...... An astonishing achievement that you have achieved to adjust yourself so well and so intensely to get well ... ... That is exactly the way that will make you get well again ... ... well and free ... ... on the outside but also on the inside ... ... You can use the opportunity today to adjust your entire organism even more to it ... ... to align all your senses with your body can finally come to rest and recover again ... ... That depends today and you adjust yourself with all your strength ... ... you direct all your positive thoughts and wishes towards this one goal ... ... get well ... ... so well and so quickly as possible ... ... get well ... ... as good and as quickly as possible ... ... and that is much easier than you thought ... ... The loving wishes are much easier than the arduous struggle that you have had for so long......you are already fighting ... ... Now, in this state of calm and relaxation, it is the honest and intense desire that can develop ... ... the desire for healing and freedom ... ... the desire for relief from pain and difficulties and for the freedom that then occurs... ... and you succeed very well, this wish so honestly and with such conviction to feel that your organism is clearly preparing to use all of its energy and strength.....collect in order to actually get well ... ... faster than you thought ... ... because now it is to feel the necessary calm ... ... Now in this calm, your body has the time and energy that it needs to require ... ... But there is still more possible ... ... You have thought for so long about which connections can cure diseases and which give them breeding ground ... ... You know that the battle of your mind was often preoccupied with so many things that you weren't free enough to take care of yourself ... ... Now it should be different ... ... now it is different ... ... Now it comes on you ... ... Now you allow yourself to rest ... ... Now you allow yourself to be very important...... you put yourself at the center of your life...... you are now the most important person in your life...... you allow your body to come to rest...... you allow your body now to devote all of its strength and energy to itself ... ... This thought fills you in completely ... ... the thought of allowing your body to be all around you, to take care of yourself ... ... It is really remarkable how much you manage to spread exactly this thought completely in your organism ... ... to give space to this thought of yourself in your body ... ... to give space in your soul to this thought of yourself...... You feel into yourself...... You can already feel the change if you concentrate entirely on your body ... ... You feel the relaxation as a signal that your body may now only be for itself and may be there for itself ... ... with your permission, with your loving permission ... ... your body uses this freedom to get well... ... as fast and as good as it can ... ... your body uses this freedom with your permission ... ...because your permission is necessary and helpful ... ... and you give it again to your thoughts ... ... you are completely prepared to say: I allow my body to become healthy... ... now ... ... I allow my body to get healthy ... ... now ...... That's the right way to do it...... you're doing it right...... because you've always wanted to be healthy, get healthy and stay healthy ... ... you know today that it helps you to actively deal with it ... ... to actively adjust to it and now officially you allow yourself to get healthy ... ... because that is the loving signal to your organism, the greatest strength and the most of the energy ... ... on healing ... ... on getting well ... ...for being healthy ... ... Today you allow it ... ... even more, you decide that it has to be ...... You arrange it ... ... All strength is now for you ... ... Everything else can wait; now your health comes up ... ... only on your health ... ... the power to heal is there ... ... it belongs to you ... ... and your body now only uses it for you, until you are healthy again and you are satisfied ... ... as healthy as possible ... ... as satisfied as possible ... ... as healthy as possible ... ... as satisfied as possible ... ... Your permission is what your body has now understood ... ... really amazing how quickly you have implemented this idea of getting well within yourself ... ... really amazing how quickly your body has understood this message... ... this request ... ... this instruction to be able to use all your strength to recover ... ...and actually to use ... ... your strength for you ... ... all your strength only for you, because you need them most now ... ... To give your body even more security ... ... even more of the feeling that it is actually only be allowed to take care of you ... ... you say it again very clearly in your mind ... ...You say: Yes, I allow myself to use my strength only for myself ... ... Yes, I allow myself, to put my healing in the foreground now ... ... Yes, I allow myself to be healthy again, like that fast and as good as possible...... Yes, I allow myself to be healthy again, as fast and as well as possible ... ...

You memorize this sentence, which will become the principle of your life ... ... Yes, I take the liberty of doing it again to be healthy as quickly and as well as possible ... ... And every day you remind yourself of these permission that you have given yourself ... ... to this promise that you have made to yourself ... ... Yes, I do allow myself to be healthy again, as quickly and as well as I can ... ... Every morning when you get up you say this sentence ... ... Yes, I allow myself to be healthy again, as quickly and as well as possible... ... and immediately you prepare yourself to do exactly that ... ... Yes, I allow myself, to be healthy again, as quickly and as well as possible ... ...

#2

You know that there are many connections between getting sick ... ... whatever exactly caused your illness or caused the most, there are many factors that play a role with getting well ... ... You know how difficult it was often in everyday life, to take care of yourself ... ... to be there for yourself and to calm down ... ... the fastest healing is always possible if we can take the time for ourselves ... ... that was not always possible in the past...... This is how stresses have accumulated that like heavy loads are on and in you and have cost a lot of strength ... ... Now it is time to let go as many burdens as possible in order to become lighter again ... ... and to be able to become and just to get better ... ... you have internalized this thought, the thought of getting well again and getting better if you are more relaxed inside ... ... But that's easy to say ... ... Worries and burdens don't just go away when we want it that way ... ... But that is not necessary at all ... ... What is more important is that the stresses and worries that you have had and have, moving away from your illness ... ... That is possible ... ... Your inner being knows that ... which often prevent us from getting well ... ... the unresolved conflicts ... ... the old anger... ... the unspoken anger ... ... the many disappointments in life ... ... if we succeed in taking a closer look at them or at least recognizing that they prevent us from becoming healthy, then we can remove them from our illness ... ... the old burdens we can then solve it later or work on it in our thoughts ... ... we can use our old ones accept feelings, because they help us to get well ... ... even and especially when it is exhausting and arduous feelings... ... feelings never make us sick, only the repression of feelings ... ... So today you are completely prepared for it, all the burdens from the sick place or from that to detach the sick area of your body in order to send them back into the world of your feelings ... ...there they help you to understand yourself and to become healthy ... ... The releasing of the old feelings and the old burdens from your body are actually possible as soon as you focus on the let in thoughts that you can control that yourself ... ... and you have this let in thought... ... amazing how much this thought completely fulfills you... ... the thought of detaching problems from your body ... ... putting burdens in your emotional world back there in order to process them as feelings ... ... burdens of your thoughts, of your mind, to put them back there in order to process them with your mind and in your to solve thoughts ... ... your body has nothing to do with it ... ... because you decide that...... You make it clear to yourself that your body did not become ill voluntarily, it just happened...... Nobody is to blame for it...... But it can be changed, your body can use his strength for himself ... ... As soon as the feelings and thoughts return to their own place, your body will succeed better and faster in approaching itself... ... He does it that way, but so far he has also needed a lot of strength for the feelings and the repressed thoughts ... ... But now everything is different ... ... Now everything is different ... ... You liberate your body ... ... now ... ... you liberate your body ... ... now ... ... First, loosen up the feelings that do not belong to your illness ... ... all unseen feelings that are in the sick place, peel off and flow back into your organism and become too feelings, that you can feel again ... ... maybe that feels strange at first, like a tingling sensation or like warmth or cold ... ... because you feel that something is actually changing inside of you ... ... that your body is freed from old feelings ... ... and angers are released from your body ... ... anger are completely released from your body - now! ... [Allow what feels like half a minute, and then read on.] ...... Grief and disappointment dissolve from your body ... ... grief and disappointment dissolve completely out of your body - now! ... [Allow what feels like half a minute, and then read on.] ...... Helplessness and fear dissolve from your body ... ... helplessness and fear dissolve completely and even out of your body - now! ... [Allow what feels like half a minute, and then read on.] ... ... Despair and hopelessness dissolve from your body ... ... Despair and hopelessness dissolve completely from your body - now! ... [What felt like half a minute leave, and then read on.] ... Then thoughts of worries and difficulties detach themselves from your body too to relieve ... ... The thoughts go back to your mind, because there they can be resolved ... ... only there ... ...thoughts of worries in the family dissolve from your body ... ... thoughts of worries in the family are completely detached from your body - now! ... [Allow what feels like half a minute to then read on.] .. Thoughts of professional and financial problems loosen from your body...... thoughts to solve professional and financial problems completely from your body - now! ... [One allows

what feels like half a minute, and then read on.]... ......
Thoughts about the worries that you know best from your life are released from your body ... ... thoughts about the worries that you know best from your life dissolve completely and even out of your body - now! ... [Allow what feels like half a minute, and then read on.] ...

Again and again feelings and thoughts detach themselves from the illness of your body when you adjust yourself internally to do it ... ... every day you tell yourself: I free my body from old ones feelings and old thoughts ... ... and even at night when you sleep, this thought is in you and works in you ... ... I free my body from old feelings and old thoughts ... ...Now! ... ...

#3

The following variant of a hypnosis main part works with a physical anchor in the form of a targeted touching of the diseased body area or the diseased area with your own hand. An anchor is a trigger that is supposed to create a certain feeling or arouse a certain thought. We want to help the client to get well and to heal by "laying on of hands" as constructive an inner attitude as possible. For this we go in four steps forward. First of all, it is important to initiate a deep state of relaxation with the help of suggestions. Select the appropriate procedures and texts for this introduction, consolidation and compliance. In the second step we help the client, one if possible to adopt positive and constructive beliefs. In the third step we put our hand as an anchor on the diseased area of the body, provided that it is not in the intimate zone. Discuss in any case, beforehand, whether it is okay for the client to put your hand on his body. If not, skip this step. In the fourth step, the client uses his own hand as an anchor on the diseased area of his body. Our hand that as "Therapist's hand" is usually seen as more effective in the subjective belief of the client, it transfers the "healing power" to the client's hand. This approach is probably very rarely used outside of energetic healing work, but I would like to expressly encourage all therapists to try it out. This is not about energetic laying on of hands, but can also be combined with it. Try it out - the effect will speak for itself!

Now come even deeper to rest ... ... Imagine that you could sink into yourself as in one very soft pillows ... ... with every breath you sink deeper into yourself ... ... dive into them infinite depth of your thoughts ... ... into the infinite depth of your feelings ... ... into the infinite depth of peace and security ... ... with every breath, every time you exhale, you go deeper into relaxation ... ... and deeper ... ... [in the rhythm of the breath of the client, please, the word "deeper" exactly speaking while exhaling and stretching a little longer than the client's actual exhalation. That causes suction into a deeper trance.] ... ... deeper and deeper ... ... deeper ... ... deeper ... ... deeper...... That's the way it is...... deep calm creates new strength to get well...... that lies in calm strength ... ... it is actually true ... ... strength lies in rest ... ... that lies in rest possibility of quick healing ... ... faster healing … … better healing … … even the miraculous healing … … It is always more possible than what we believe … … always more than we believe … … Today it is important to make everything possible that you have been up to now………maybe you haven't really been able to believe … … or you haven't really imagined it yet … … today it works … … here and today … … .. … Now imagine the word healing … … You sees it in bold letters in front of yours inner eye…… healing…… thick black letters on a light background…… In bold letters you can see the word healing … … Concentrate on it and keep reading it again … … healing … … This word takes up all of your thoughts, you only think this one word … … you only see this one word … …. Just feel this one word … … healing… … So your body adjusts itself to it with all its might at this very moment, just like that to create quickly and as best as possible now … … healing … … Then you imagine that this word moves through your body … … you can put it anywhere in or on yours……..Let the body appear … … So you will also find the word healing in / on …[sick spot or zone or call it an organ] … There is the word healing … … So you can feel this even more clearly, I now put my hand on this spot … … I now touch you very gently with my hand ... ... [Place one hand flat and gently on the diseased area] ... ... now you feel some warmth there too ... ... The warmth that you feel now, where my hand is, shows you that the word healing, which you have placed there, is beginning to work ... ...now direct all your mindfulness to this place and feel my hand ... ... feel right there too your body ... ... feel the warmth right there ... ... feel the effect of the right there too healing ... ... just like that ... ... That's right ... ... This is how it works best ... ... Concentrate further on this spot ... ... [Wait what feels like half a minute, then read on] ... ... My hand for your body is a signal to activate the word healing at this point ... ... my hand is a signal to your body that now all power of self-healing is activated ... ... so intensely and so as strong as possible ... ... right now! ... ... your body is imprinted on it, your whole organism this is imprinted ... ... my hand becomes a sign of healing ... ... Now I take my hand away again and then you can put your own hand there and feel that you can also feel the warmth of healing ... ... I take my hand now back...... [Slowly pulling your hand away]...... Now put your own hand on this spot...... [Briefly wait. If the client does not comply with the request, ask again a little more clearly or if necessary lead the hand of the client, with the words ... I'll help you something, grab your wrist and take your hand and lead it to the sick spot ...] ... ... Now you can feel your own hand on your body ... ... your body knows that this is a signal for it to place the word healing where it is. You can feel the hand ... ... and the warmth that you can feel right at this point or now, shows you that the healing effect begins at this very moment ... ...direct your attention to the contact between your hand and your body and feel the warmth there...... very intense...... concentrate on this spot...... your body saves it...... your whole organism saves it...... your organism knows that the healing effect must always come into play when you put your hand on this area... ... or on another part of your body affected by illness ... ... your hand is for your body a signal to activate the word healing at this point ... ... your hand is a signal to your body that now all power of self-healing is activated ... ... so intensely and so as strong as possible ... ... right now! ... ... your body is imprinted on it, your whole organism memorize ... ... your hand becomes a sign of healing ... ...

Whenever you put your hand on your body, this is the signal for your organism to activate self-healing power and to enable healing ... ... like now ... ... just like now ... ... every day you can help yourself by lying down and coming to rest and then put your own hand on your body ... ... your organism then immediately makes its entire self-healing power available and your healing begins

#4

The following variant of a main part of hypnosis works with a physical anchor in the form of a targeted touch of the diseased body zone or the diseased area with one's own hand, which is "charged" beforehand by touching a healthy area. An anchor is a trigger that is supposed to create a certain feeling or arouse a certain thought. We want to help the client by "laying on of hands" in an inner as constructive a way as possible Attitude towards getting well and healing. We do this in four steps in front. First of all, it is important to achieve a deep state of relaxation with the help of suggestions initiate. To do this, select the appropriate procedures and texts for the introduction, in-depth study and compliance. In the second step, we help the client to be as positive as possible and to adopt a constructive belief system. In the third step, the client puts a hand as anchor on a healthy area of the body, preferably in an easily accessible area upper body. With the help of suggestions he should imagine that the hand would be healthy state. In the fourth step, the client puts the same hand as an anchor on the diseased area of his body. The hand should transport the healthy feeling there. Also this approach may sound unusual, or perhaps even esoteric, but it has nothing to do with it. It is important that the client anchor the idea that the healthy parts and areas of his body can support or heal the sick areas! I have used this approach very often, and never before had a client found it unusual!

Now come even deeper to rest ... ... Imagine that you could sink into yourself as in one very soft pillows ... ... with every breath you sink deeper into yourself ... ... dive into them infinite depth of your thoughts ... ... into the infinite depth of your feelings ... ... into the infinite depth of peace and security ... ... with every breath, every time you exhale, you go deeper into relaxation ... ... and deeper ... ... [in the rhythm of the breath of the client, please, the word "deeper" exactly speaking while exhaling and stretching a little longer than the client's actual exhalation. That causes suction into a deeper trance.] ... ... deeper and deeper ... ... deeper ... ... deeper ... ... deeper...... That's the way it is...... deep calm creates new strength to get well...... that lies in calm strength ... ... it is actually true ... ... strength lies in rest ... ... that lies in rest possibility of quick healing ... ... faster healing ... ... better healing ... ... even the miraculous healing ... ... It is always more possible than what we believe ... ... always more than we believe ... ... Today it is important to make everything possible that you have been up to now and maybe you haven't really been able to believe ... ... or you haven't really imagined it yet ... ... today it works ... ... here and today ... ... Now concentrate on a part of your body that is completely healthy and now at this moment, feels good ... ... you should be able to reach the spot easily with your hand, because it is important that you actually touch them with your hand right away ... ... [It is best to speak yourself a position that you agreed with the client before starting the hypnosis. Explain briefly the process before it starts, this makes work easier and avoids clumsiness.]...... Feel yourself into this spot and feel how good it feels ... ... how nice it is at this point to be healthy and to feel it too ... ... This area feels good ... ... really healthy... ... You imagine that this is how your whole body should feel ... ... and that you feel and use the energy from healthy areas of your body to heal diseased areas ...... You put your right / left hand on this healthy area... [Choose the hand with which the healthy area is easiest to reach and address the area directly]... with it you can feel the feeling even more clearly ... ... The warmth that you feel now, where yours hand is, shows you that your hand is fully connected with the feeling of healthy energy in you...... Now direct all your mindfulness to this point and feel your hand ... ... feel right there your body too...... feel the warmth right there too...... feel the energy right there too the healing ... ... just like that ... ... that's the way it is ... ... this is how it works best ... ... concentrate continue on this point ... ... [wait what feels like half a minute, then read on] ... ... your hand absorbs the entire information of the healing power in you and can transport it ... ... Really amazing that it's so easy to do ... ... and really amazing how good your hand actually picks up this information in order to transport it ... ... so your hand can transport information about healing from outside ... ... no internal blockages or obstacles stand in the way ... ... Now take your hand and put it where the disease is ... ... [Better the one in question speak directly to ... Put your hand on your stomach now ... ... Wait a moment. If the client does not comply with the request, ask again a little more clearly or, if necessary, guide the client's hand with the words ... I'll help you a little, grab your wrist and take your hand and guide it...]...... Now you feel your hand on your body again...... You feel the warmth between your hand and your body and know that this is a sign of the connection ... ... your body knows that this is a signal for it to release the healthy and healing energy now wherever the hand can be felt ... ... and the warmth that you can feel at this point shows you that in this very moment the healing effect begins ... ... direct your attention of the contact between your hand and your body and feel the warmth there ... ... very intensely ... ... concentrate on this point ... ... your body takes the power of its healthy parts now to get healthy again ... ... your whole organism saves it ... ... Your organism knows that the healing effect must always come into its own when you put your hand on this area ... ... or on any other sick area of your body ... ... your body imprints it, your whole organism imprints it ... ... your hand becomes a sign of healing ... ...

Consolidation (post-hypnotic assignment)

Anytime you put your hand on your body, on something that feels good, this will be the signal for your organism to absorb the healthy and healing energy ... ... if you then moving the same hand to a place affected by illness or pain or discomfort is affected ... ... then your hand gives the healing energy to precisely this move, so it can get well again ... ... Every day you can help yourself by lying down and resting and then placing your own hand on a healthy area of your body and then on a sick one ... ... Your organism then immediately restores it and the entire self-healing power is available and your healing begins ... ...

#5

You are here today to do something for yourself and for the healing of your illness ... [If possible address the disease directly ... the healing of your stomach ulcer, etc. ...] ... ... you already have done a lot, you received treatments, tried to behave yourself like the fastest possible recovery can take place...... body and mind are closely linked...... One says man says: Sana in corpora sano, which means something like living in a healthy body and a healthy mind ... ... and in fact mind and body are related ... ... or more precisely thoughts and body reactions...... also feelings and body reactions...... and maybe you know, yes, that thoughts and ideas in us are reactions to deep feelings ... ... we also use our inner images and ideas, visualizations, and our feeling influence ... ... help ourselves to get into a constructive emotional state and this in an attitude of getting well ... ... We can change into a healing mode with inner images ... ... That is actually possible and you can do it too ... ... The real one challenge here is to keep creating constructive images in us and to keep it upright ... ... In everyday life we do not always and not permanently succeed ... ... but in a state of calm ... ... in a state of trance, it is much easier for us ... ... here and now so you can do a lot for yourself, a lot for your healing mode ... ... and if it does, here you can turn it on, then it will also be much easier in your everyday life and if you want, every day ... ... First we start by clearing your mind ... ... all disturbing thoughts now you let go ... ... Imagine a little white light that shines inside you ... ... You find it in your imagination and see it in your mind's eye, so in your imagination ... ... you are illuminated directly by this white light, like a lamp hanging over you ... ... Let this light get brighter and brighter and allow the white light to clear your thoughts now ... ... all disturbing thoughts pass in the white light ... ... the white light is getting brighter, you stand in a cone of light that surrounds your whole body ... ... and with your permission the white light cleanses your thoughts and feelings ... ... you let go all thoughts ... ... that goes by itself, you don't have to do anything special for it ... ... just leave the white light there and develop its cleansing effect ... ... your thoughts become free ... ... you let them just come and go ... ... keep opening up to new thoughts and new feelings ...... White light surrounds you and makes you free from all disturbing thoughts and feelings ... ... You relax deeper and deeper ... ... and deeper and deeper ... ... All thoughts that are involved, all having dealt with disease and therapy now, move on and simply dissolve in the white light... ... Isn't it wonderful that the idea of white light actually ends your thoughts ...... And isn't it really surprising that you find yourself thinking about white light and you feel free and actually you are free? ...... Really astonishing, but it works...... you feel it and can experience it for yourself ... ... you succeed ... ... you succeed in particular ... ... you succeed it now ... ...Now you can switch to the healing mode ... ... To do this, imagine a golden light, that shines down on you from above ... ... A golden cone of light surrounds you and closes your whole body ...... a golden light as a source of healing...... and with this golden light you switch to the healing mode ... ... in this state , healing can place ... ... faster than usual...... better than usual...... more sustainable than usual...... golden light activated your self-healing power ... ... you may even feel a change ... ... already now ... ... maybe a tingling sensation in your body ... ... some warmth or it gets cool ... ... or one part of your body just feels different than a few minutes ago ... ... but maybe you want just continue to enjoy the idea of the light and don't even think about all that ...... Then just stay with the idea of golden light activating your healing mode and keep going constructively for you ... ... Look at the light in front of your inner eye ... ... Look how it glitters and sparkles ... ... golden light of healing ... ... Isn't it wonderful that the idea of golden light actually drives your recovery? ... ... and it isn't really amazing that at the idea of golden light you can and actually make you feel free...........are you free ?...... Really amazing, but it works...... You feel it and can experience it for yourself... ... you succeed ... ... you succeed in particular ... ... you succeed now ... ... imagine further pretend that you are surrounded by the golden light ... ... [Wait what feels like half a minute, then continue read] ... ... Now let the light go away ... ... Just turn it off in your imagination and introduce yourself at the same time that you have now absorbed so much of the golden light that your body shines golden ... ... your arms ... ... your legs ... ... your stomach ... ... your hands and your feet ... ... your whole body shines and glitters golden ... ... in your imagination that is very simple, but it is more than just an idea ... ... deep within you, this very idea is linked to an important step ... ... the change and remaining in the healing mode ... ...

And every day you can do something for your recovery ... ... You simply give yourself a time of the calm and mindfulness, lay down or sit down comfortably and close your eyes ... ... Then take your imagine, how white light surrounds you and immediately you feel the cleansing and liberating effect again ... ... Immediately you will be free of all thoughts ... ... Then you imagine golden light...... Whenever you imagine golden light, you switch to your healing mode ... ... into that state that can help you the most to get well as quickly and as well as possible ...... to get well as quickly and as well as possible ... ... like now ... ... just like now ... ..

#6

You have already dealt a lot with the question of psychosomatics … …you have thought about what connections there are between the psyche and getting sick … … maybe you have also asked yourself why you got sick … … thought about the conditions and contexts that contributed to it in you … … you have already asked yourself a lot of questions … … and because there is a connection between soul and body or between psyche and body you are here … … that's why you're looking for help in hypnosis / psychotherapy … … so I want you to take your question seriously; the connections between your psyche and your illness and more yet, I want to share it with you to promote your recovery … … I want you for this, invite you to pursue a similar and perhaps a completely different question today … … one question that deals just as intensively with the relationship between psyche and body … …The question you have asked so far is: What does my psyche have to cause my illness? … … today I want to offer you the question: What can my psyche do for my recovery?... ... because your psyche, your thoughts and your feelings can add something to contribute to your recovery ... ... They can help you to be as constructive as possible... ... deep inside, in the areas that you cannot simply control with your will... ... an even more constructive attitude can arise there ... ... It is helpful if the belief in the disease is dissolved ... ... Over time we get used to diseases and in the case of long-lasting illnesses in particular, we then at least partially believe that the cure will no longer succeed ... ... what your psyche can contribute to your recovery is the dissolving of these thoughts that are clinging to the illness without you wanting to ... ... And for that you can use your imagination ... ... because you just can't determine what should happen inside you, but you can visualize it and this inform your body and your psyche what to do ... ... images come in the depths of your feelings much easier than wishes or commands ... ... your inner images, the images of your imagination, make truth in your subconscious ... ... and that might be easier than you thought... So let's start with ... ... In your imagination there is a place of recovery ... ... An in this place you are now ... ... at the place of your recovery ... ... Your illness is here as a thick rock ... ... It lies directly in front of you … … you look at the stone and concentrate completely on it … … it is the inner image of your illness … … the illness that you can change with your inner images … … you know that there are inner blockages… … blockages that are in our feelings … … you could find them and fathom them … … yes you can do something that is easier and faster … … you can turn to yourself …… with mindfulness and respect … … and love from you, for yourself … … you just turn to your feelings … … but maybe you are wondering how you can best do it … … just concentrate on the image of the rock in front of you … … direct all of your attention to this stone and with it your mindfulness on your feelings … … it works by itself… … The more you succeed in concentrating on the image of this stone lump, the more you turn to your feelings in your mindfulness … … don't think about it … …thoughts cannot capture feelings … … Mindfulness and concentration are more than enough… … you don't need more … … Imagine the boulder … …… … And imagine that little pieces of him break off slowly … … with every breath … …whenever you exhale, the wind of your breath blows towards the stone and loosens a few small pieces from him … … At first it may be small pieces, like grains of sand so big, that trickle down from him ... ... With each exhalation, some sand loosens and trickles to the ground ... ... Look at the stone and imagine it ... ... Let this picture emerge clearly in front of your inner eye, because with it you connect with your feelings and detach them from the illness ... ... just like you do individually detaching pieces of stone ... ... Breathe consciously and observe more and more in your imagination of sand is crumbling from the stone ... ... a little more with every breath ... ... with every breath a little more ... ... and over time the loosened pieces get bigger ... ... and the big chunk out stone, which stands for your illness, becomes smaller ... ... smaller with every breath ... ... with each one single breath smaller ... ... smaller and smaller ... ... keep concentrating on this picture ... ... The clearer you let this picture become in front of your inner eye, the more this connection between inner blockages and being ill will dissolve ... ... and that is exactly what helps you to get well ...... All blockages that could be in your feelings and thoughts, you can edit there also and take care of ... ... but today you first really release them from being ill... ... This is what you can do for your recovery ... ... Imagine the picture further and leave that stone get smaller and smaller because with every breath another piece of it falls away ... ... until it has become very small and at some point dissolves completely ... ...

Your inner being has long since understood this trick and knows that it actually works like this ... ...faith moves mountains, they say, but strictly speaking, it's the inner images, the mountains be able to move and dissolve boulders ... ... first in your imagination and then also in your waking life ... ... you can intensify that ... ... just imagine in the evening, briefly before falling asleep the boulders of illness again ... ... and then in sleep, in a state of calm, your breathing ensures that the image dissolves ... ... and with it the way for that to get well.

#7

Ide motoric skills describe the phenomenon that our body follows our feelings and thoughts with movements. In everyday life, this consequence shows up as a person's posture, muscle tension and movement patterns, which naturally change with mood and thoughts. In trance ide motoric signals can be used to obtain information that the client is not actively involved in communication. The subconscious can, for example, ask questions with an agreed finger signal. Of course, ide motoric reactions can also be used suggestively, for example in arm levitations and catalepsies. Such an approach, which I will also use in the following text apply, strengthens the trust in the hypnosis and in one's own ability to change and thus promotes the therapy. To do this, hold the client's arm by the wrist and pull it diagonally upwards, without to hyperextend the arm. During the gesture to hold, test whether the arm is by giving way slightly is already being held cataleptically and release it as soon as the catalepsy is over.

You know that it is emotional and mental burdens that can keep you from getting well...... The other way around, it is possible to cure or alleviate illnesses that becomes much faster, the more you manage to get rid of these burdens ... ... Perhaps you also think that it would be not really easy ... ... but it's easier than you think ... ... I'll show you how to do it and how to do it all... ... here and today ... ... I'll show you today how to do it ... ... you even you can do it deep inside of you ... ... your inner being can do that ... ... and it can also show you as soon as it is, has done that ... ... For this we use your arm ... ... because your insides ... ... your subconscious can show you with your arm as soon as it has deposited the disturbing loads ... ...[Now the client's arm is held by the therapist until the catalepsy is gone. Discuss please do the procedure before the session with the client and cancel any contact during the trance always immediately. Always avoid fright or defensive reactions!] ... ... I'll take your wrist and hold your arm for you ... ... Just let it go ... ... Everything happens for your own good ... ... I will help you to lay off your inner burdens now and thus free yourself for relief and healing ... ... [Now hold the client's arm by the wrist and pull it diagonally upwards, without to hyperextend the arm. During the subsequent postural suggestion, test whether the arm is already being held cataleptically by gently giving in and release it as soon as the catalepsy is over.] ... ... watch your arm now. It gets tighter and tighter, as tight as an iron bar ... ... and at the same time as light as a feather ... ... so it's very easy to hold your arm ... ... hold it up as if it were held by an invisible balloon ... ... your arm is getting tighter ... ... always, always firmer, very firm and stable ... ... your arm assumes position and remains in exactly this position... ... Your arm becomes stiff and firm and stays in exactly this position ... ... It is light and very firm ... ... your arm is completely immobile and rigid ... ... completely immobile and rigid ... ... your arm remains in exactly this position ... ... just like that ... ... [possibly. lengthen it a little if the arm is not held, but this should happen quickly. For clients, the cataleptic state is not a subjective burden or effort. He has the feeling that the arm will hold by itself.] Now I give your subconscious the task of today to lay off the inner burdens so that you can become healthy ... ... they become meaningless for your body ... ... your body becomes free from these burdens, also and especially when you think about them and your feeling

...... your inner being arranges the loads in such a way that your body becomes free of them ... ...Your arm shows you how much your subconscious has already achieved ... ...Your arm is now slowly moving again and slowly sinks onto the surface ... ... That goes in exactly the same time it takes your subconscious to remove all of your stresses...... Your arm is now mobile and sinks down and as soon as the arm rises and arrives the pad, all thoughts and worries for your body have become insignificant ... ... As soon as your arm touches the pad, you feel physically liberated and your body can become healthy ... ... you liberate your body ... ... now ... ... you liberate your body ... ... now ... . [Wait until the arm sinks onto the surface. This can take a while, but it can also be quick. The speed does not play a role in the success. It is a reflection of how firm the will to change and how great any doubts there may be. Just let it go as it happens. Should the arm does not move, please help with the following or similar suggestions.] Take your time ... ... do this at your own pace ... ... at your own pace ... ... As soon as the time is right, your arm will move too ... ... Surely today is the right day for it, then your arm will move right away ... ...If today is not the right day, then your arm will not move today, but today it does, because it is the right day, it will also move soon ... ...Your body is now completely free of your mental and emotional burdens and feels free ... ... completely free ... ... stress and worries are meaningless for your body ... ...your body can feel good and relaxed ... ... your body can get healthy ... ... now

#8

You have often heard that you are sick ... ... maybe you have already said that yourself it would be so, because there is this disease ... ... But today it depends, the whole thing to take a closer look ... ... to distinguish between your body, which is this disease in itself and your soul, which is not sick ... ... Only your body is sick, you are healthy ... ... Perhaps it seems to you as if it were the same, but that's not true ... ... You are not your body ... ... You only live in it ... ... So you have a sick part, your body ... ... and a healthy part and that is you ... ... You are healthy and you can help your body, too to get well again ... ... as healthy as you are very deep in your soul ... ... so use it now, your common mind ... ... your healthy thoughts ... ... and your healthy attention ... ... focus your attention on the sick part of your body ... . [Please address the sick body, the sick organ or the sick area directly. Always call the illness "illness... of your body to make it clear that the mental or emotional part is healthy and does not belong to the disease ... ... Example: Pay attention to the stomach ulcer in your body ...]

… … give your body as much attention and mindfulness as possible … … feel into the sick part of your body … [Better the sick part, the sick organ or the sick address the area directly.] … and imagine that you can send the wind of your breath there… … Imagine that the air you breathe flows through your nose into the airways … … you are good at that feel, because you feel the air you breathe through your nostrils … … and imagine them flowing into your lungs … … You can feel that too, because your upper body rises during the inhale … … And now imagine that you could flow the air you breathe into any part of your body, let it in … … simply through the lungs and then further into your body … … exactly to that sick area … So now and with the next breaths you breathe exactly there … … exactly to … [sick spot, address the diseased organ or the diseased area directly.] … excellent … … you do it well …… that's the way it is right … … continue to breathe exactly there … … very close to … [sick spot, sick one, address the organ or the sick area directly.] …… … Now you may already feel the beneficial effect of your breath in your body, because healing calm arises … … maybe you already feel it … … or maybe a little later … … But you can achieve a lot more … … You can get all the blockages and all the incrustations there to solve ... ... all the stresses and strains of your life that are in you with the disease had put your body into it ... ... This also works with your breathing ... ... Breathe on to exactly this important part of your body ... ... your healthy thoughts now direct the inner power of healing ... ... your healthy creativity now directs the inner power of healing ... ... your healthy part now directs the inner power of healing ... ...The wind of your breath envelops the disease in your body and, with the exhalation, let it go out ... ... The wind of your breath envelops the illness in your body and with the exhalation you exhale the illness ... ... Concentrate on your breathing, because with everyone exhale you let something out ... ... with every breath you can free yourself from something ... ... and the liberation helps your body to get well ... ...[Now please stay exactly in the client's breathing rhythm and always speak the following suggestions while the client exhales. Make sure you breathe out clearly, so speak exhale the suggestion with a deep exhalation.]...... [Client exhales]... You exhale, letting anger and anger escape...... [Client exhales]... once again ... ... [Wait for another "empty" breath, without suggestion, then take the next oneContinue suggestion] ... ... [Client exhales]... You exhale and let all disappointments escape...... [Client breathes off] ... again ... [wait for another breath, then continue with the next suggestion]...... [Client exhales]... You exhale and let unfulfilled longing escape...... [Client breathes off] ... again ... [wait for another breath, then continue with the next suggestion]...... [Client exhales]... You exhale, letting out all guilt feelings...... [Client breathes off] ... again ... [wait for another breath, then continue with the next suggestion]...... [Client exhales]... You exhale and let go of the illness...... [Client exhales]... You exhale and let go of the illness...... [Client exhales]... You exhale and let go the illness....Come on ... ...Your body adjusts itself more and more intensely, with every conscious inhalation the disease enveloping your body, capturing it ... ... and then letting go with the exhalation ... ... with every breath a piece of it ... ... So you can consciously and purposefully every day work to relieve the disease and rid your body of it ... ... Whenever you go into a state of calm and resolve to help your body, you breathe very consciously ... [address the sick area, organ or the sick area directly.] ... and breathe everything out. ... ...

like today ... ... just like today ... ... You can do it, you have just made it that way ... ...

#9

You have dealt extensively with your illness, perhaps you have understood how illness develops and how it can be cured ... ... how long it takes and how much effort it can cost ... ... You know that you are in your thoughts and even more so in your feelings, you can do a lot to help yourself get better ... ... and as long as the illness is still there, in enduring and in dealing with it ... ... There is healing above all in the world of our feelings, because emotions can be very powerful ... ... I will help you today, to mobilize as much as possible of your own healing power, of your self-healing power ... ... Strictly speaking, the self-healing power does not need to be mobilized because it is always active ... ... but sometimes it is helpful to remove everything that is disturbing ...... the disturbing thing that can slow it down ... ... But today you can speed it up again ... ... you prepare yourself for an inner journey ... ... a journey to a far-away land, which at the same time is completely close ... ... the land of your dreams ... ... feel the rhythm of your breathing and follow it ... ... with the wind of your breath you leave your thoughts and go to the land of dreams ... ... You stand on a wide path and just go ... ... You let your feelings guide you and follow this path that seems familiar to you ... ... You have been walking on it for a long time, without you actually know...... Then you will see a sign at the edge of the path that says "Path your illness "... ... So you are walking the path of illness ... ... Illness is already preoccupying you long that your thoughts are now far too busy with her ... ... sometimes that was necessary, because you have also taken care of treatment ... ... you have the way found here ... ... But then again it was too much ... ... you could hardly do anything to undertake different things and think of something else, your strength was so absorbed by the illness ... ... The path leads you into a forest, into the forest of your thoughts ... ... Often you have the feeling that you can no longer sort your thoughts, maybe also the wish to get out of the constant rush of thoughts ... ... to take a break ... ... finally relief to find ... ... But like the tall trees around you are in this forest and so make it dark and impenetrable, your thoughts often stand on you like obstacles path ... ... Then you decide to simply leave this path ... ... Here in the land of yours dreams it is very easy ... ... You just walk down the path and just follow your feelings or your mood ... ... walk through the trees ... ... on the soft forest floor ...... Then you notice that the forest is much easier to penetrate than you thought ... ... the further you go and as more you move away from the old path, the lighter and lighter the forest becomes ... ... You take a deep breath...... Then you come to a small lake in the forest...... a small waterfall brings fresh water into the lake and a stream lets the water flow away again...... So now flows constantly fresh water in this beautiful forest lake ... ... you look up ... ... the sun shines and falls directly onto the lake ... ... He invites you to a bath ... ... and because it is so beautiful and warm and you can use relaxation so well, take off your clothes and walk in the small lake for swimming ... ... the water is pleasant, just as you like it ... ... you lay down in the water and make yourself comfortable ... ... you enjoy bathing in the land of dreams, and that it is a healing bath for your body ... ...The water is crystal clear and pure...... You look at the waterfall and see that the falling water glitters and sparkles...... It looks like thousands of little stars. ... Little golden lights that spread throughout the water ... ...This golden power strengthens your body ... ... The little golden lights are attracted from your body as if by a magnet ... ... They slip through your skin and into your body and give you a pleasant feeling ... ... a thousand little golden lights heal your body in the land of dreams ... ... You see how they slip under your skin and continue inside shine ... ... you give yourself peace and serenity ... ... you trust that the golden lights will help you to get healthy ... ... you stay in the water and enjoy the healing bath ... ... You dream of what it will be like as soon as your body is completely healthy again ...... You imagine how free you will be again ... ... and you enjoy the bath in the golden lights of the dreamland ... ... Then you get out of the water and lay down in the warming sun...... You feel the golden power in you ... ... You feel that the little golden lights help you to get well ... ... You close your eyes and dream a beautiful dream of being healthy again soon...... Freed from everything that could make you sick ... ... Then you open your eyes and look on your skin ... ... There you can see the golden lights that have already done their work, out of your skin slip ... ... They rise into the sky as golden soap bubbles and take a piece of your disease with them ... ... Each light takes a small piece with it and flies in as a golden soap bubble the sky and bursts...... one golden soap bubble after the other bursts...... and with every soap bubble that bursts you become a bit more freer ... ... and healthier ... ... you follow the golden lights with your eyes and see them burst as soap bubbles ... ... the golden lights, what your body still needs to become healthy, remain in it and give you their healing power ... ... and as soon as each light has done its work, it leaves your body and flies into the heaven, where it bursts like a golden soap bubble ... ...

You know that all of this doesn't just happen in your imagination ... ... fantasy and reality are very close together ... ... sometimes both are just a blink of an eye away from each other ...... The land of dreams is just as real as the world of your everyday life ... ... You think about it, that the land of dreams is deep within you ... ... It has always been there ... ... I'm just telling you about it ...

#10

You don't just see your illness as a condition that you are at the mercy of ... ... you know that there are connections in your thoughts and in your feelings that make a accelerate disease or act as a breeding ground for it, but it can be conversely, there are opportunities to promote recovery and your own healing power ... ...because there is healing power, which we call self-healing power, in every organism, including yours...... You prepare for an inner journey...... a journey to a faraway country that is also very close at the same time...... the land of your dreams...... In this country everything is possible, even in your imagination all can happen....... And here is space just for you ... ... only for you ... ... you go to the land of dreams...... You are here to find a special medicine...... the medicine of your life...... It is so called because it comes from the experience of your life and from everything of powerful moments of your life arises ... ... even if you haven't really noticed it yet ... ...You are approaching a golden yellow cornfield ... ... In the middle of this field there are three wells like this....... This look like the fountains used to be ... ... round and made of stones ... ... with a wooden frame that carries a winch that is operated with a hand crank ... ... This is what a bucket can do, be lowered on a rope until it fills with water and then cranked up again to drink the water ... ... you go to the fountain in the cornfield ... ... you look up to the sky, which looks exactly the way you like it ... ... maybe a summer sky, if you like that ... ... maybe a stormy autumn sky ... ... or a cloudy spring sky, just as you want ... ... just so that you feel best ...... You reach the first well...... there you will find a small bottle with the inscription "Medicine of your life" ... ... it is empty ... ... But you can fill it today ... ... here and today, in the land of your dreams, create your own medicine ... ... in the world of your feelings, because there it does work for you already today ... ... You walk around the fountain and find a sign on which says "Well of your successes"...... You look into the well and see the water...... and up the surface of the water you see pictures of your own successes ... ... they rise from the depths of the well up to the surface ... ... As a child you had successes, maybe once accomplished something that you didn't think you could do yourself ... ... Maybe you climbed up a tree one day and were proud to have made it ... ... or you repaired something or dismantled something and researched ... ... a toy maybe and that too have been a success, even if it was no longer usable afterwards ... ... maybe there was success in school ...... or a particular success, an unexpectedly good grade ... ... Little by little, pictures your successes become visible ... ... successes of childhood ... ... successes of youth ... ... successes from your adult life ... ... You draw some water from the well of success with the bucket and fill a few drops in the bottle ... ... Then you go to the next well that says "Well of Overcoming" ... ... You look at the water and images arise that show you the limits that you once surmounted ... ... maybe outer limits because you have an obstacle climbed or performed a sporting performance ... ... or you were afraid of an exam and went in ... ... experienced the door of the examination room like a border ... ...like a high wall ... ... but you have overcome it ... ... and very often you also had to yourself overcome yourself ... ... overcome your inner limits ... ... your fears... ... Images rise from the depths of the well that show you what you once conquered ...... and where you had to overcome yourself ... ... many years ago ... ... in your kind at the moment ... ...

but also in yours family...... in your free time...... you draw some water from the well with a bucket the overcoming and fill a few drops into the bottle ... ... Then you go to the next one. Well that says "Well of Letting Go" ... ... You look at the water and pictures rise that show you what or whom you once had to let go ... ... Maybe you once had to letting go of good friendship ... ... It broke up or you got separated and you had to let go ... ... Perhaps you lost a valuable item or one that was just had a special value for you ... ... you could no longer find it and you had to finally let go ... ... relationships are broken in your life, you also had to let go and continue to shape your life ... ... Maybe you had to let go when someone died...... let go ... ... let go of what we have in common ... ... let go of what had happened ... ... and what you had hoped or wished to let go ... ... You had to let go of a lot ... ... That was often painful, but with each letting go there is also freedom for new things ... ... you can let go...... You have already made it so often...... You scoop some water out of the well of the overcoming with the bucket and fill a few drops into the bottle...... Then you go on and lay down on the soft ground of the cornfield ... ... You have the power of success, the power of overcoming and the power of letting go as the medicine of your own life in the small bottle that you carry with you, because you have combined your own strength into a healing medicine ...... You breathe in and out deeply...... one more time deeply in and out...... and then you drink a strong sip of the medicine of your life... ... and feel the healing effect in you ... ... at this very moment ... ...

You trust in the beneficial effects of the special medicine in the land of dreams, the land of your feelings ... ... Then you think about the fact that the land of dreams is deep inside you...... It has always been there ... ... I'm just telling you about it...

Overview of All Titles in the Series "Ten Hypnoses"

Volume 1: Smoking Cessation
Volume 2: Anxiety and Restlessness
Volume 3: Burnout
Volume 4: Reducing Overweight
Volume 5: Coping with the Past
Volume 6: Suicidal Thoughts and Attempts
Volume 7: Psycho-Oncology
Volume 8: Obsessions and Tics
Volume 9: Self-Confidence and Decision-Making
Volume 10: Grief Work
Volume 11: Psychosomatics
Volume 12: Chronic Pain
Volume 13: Depressive Thoughts
Volume 14: Panic Attacks
Volume 15: Domestic Violence, Victim Support
Volume 16: Post-Traumatic Stress
Volume 17: Exam Anxiety and Stage Fright
Volume 18: Anti-Violence Training, Offender Support
Volume 19: Addiction Tendencies
Volume 20: Social Phobia and Fear of Contact
Volume 21: Nail Biting
Volume 22: Self-Awareness and Self-Love
Volume 23: Teeth Grinding and Night Clenching
Volume 24: Feelings of Guilt
Volume 25: Fear in Crowds
Volume 26: Fear of Flying, Aviophobia
Volume 27: Fear in Enclosed Spaces, Claustrophobia
Volume 28: Tinnitus, Ear Noises
Volume 29: Fear of Heights
Volume 30: Neurodermatitis

Volume 31: Finding Inner Balance
Volume 32: Overcoming Loneliness
Volume 33: Fear of Illness, Hypochondria
Volume 34: Anticipatory Anxiety, Fear of Fear
Volume 35: Jealousy in Relationships
Volume 36: Driving Anxiety
Volume 37: New Start after Separation
Volume 38: Fear of Injections
Volume 39: Heart Anxiety Neurosis
Volume 40: Overcoming Resentment and Anger
Volume 41: Resolving Blockages and Positive Thinking
Volume 42: Stress Reduction, Stress Management
Volume 43: Body Relaxation
Volume 44: Deep Relaxation
Volume 45: Fear of the Dark
Volume 46: Falling Asleep and Staying Asleep
Volume 47: Compulsive Buying
Volume 48: Restless Legs Syndrome
Volume 49: Bulimia
Volume 50: Anorexia
Volume 51: Overcoming Nightmares
Volume 52: Imagined Deformity
Volume 53: Overcoming Distrust, Finding Trust
Volume 54: Processing Failures
Volume 55: Humiliation, Emotional Hurt
Volume 56: Distressing Compassion, Vicarious Suffering
Volume 57: Self-Forgiveness
Volume 58: Self-Awareness, Self-Confidence
Volume 59: Saying No
Volume 60: Assertiveness
Volume 61: Setting Boundaries and Self-Assertion
Volume 62: Decision-Making Ability

Volume 63: Success Orientation
Volume 64: Ruminating, Circular Thinking
Volume 65: Accepting Pregnancy
Volume 66: Birth Preparation
Volume 67: Spiritual Opening
Volume 68: Joy of Life and Inner Lightness
Volume 69: Patience and Inner Peace
Volume 70: Fibromyalgia and Rheumatism
Volume 71: Irritable Bowel Syndrome, Crohn's Disease
Volume 72: Fear of Nausea, Emetophobia
Volume 73: Stuttering and Cluttering, Speech Flow Disorders
Volume 74: Concentration and Knowledge Anchoring
Volume 75: Vitality and Spontaneity
Volume 76: Searching for Meaning and Finding Goals
Volume 77: Life Crises, Life Events
Volume 78: Workaholism, Goal Obsession
Volume 79: Helper Syndrome, Helpless Helpers
Volume 80: Medication Abuse
Volume 81: Gambling Addiction
Volume 82: Internet Addiction, Smartphone Addiction
Volume 83: Hoarding Disorder, Compulsive Collecting
Volume 84: Conspiracy Thoughts, Overvalued Ideas
Volume 85: Fear of Operations and Treatments
Volume 86: Fear of Aging
Volume 87: Travel Anxiety
Volume 88: Anxiety When Urinating, Paruresis
Volume 89: Fear of Intimacy and Togetherness
Volume 90: Fear of Blushing
Volume 91: Coming Out in Homosexuality
Volume 92: Charisma Training
Volume 93: Migraines and Chronic Headaches
Volume 94: Overcoming Allergies, Bronchial Asthma

Volume 95: Normalizing Blood Pressure
Volume 96: Compulsive Perfectionism
Volume 97: Sports Hypnosis, Motivation
Volume 98: Sports Hypnosis, Performance Enhancement
Volume 99: Determination and Focus
Volume 100: Encountering the Inner Child
Volume 101: Cravings, Binge Eating
Volume 102: Stimulating Metabolism
Volume 103: Bipolar Mood Swings
Volume 104: Borderline, Identity Crises
Volume 105: Hypomania, Euphoria, Mania
Volume 106: Restlessness, Agitation
Volume 107: Nervous Breakdown
Volume 108: Adjustment Disorders
Volume 109: Self-Alienation, Depersonalization
Volume 110: Ending Self-Pity
Volume 111: Primary Gain of Illness
Volume 112: Secondary Gain of Illness
Volume 113: Bullying, Victim Support
Volume 114: Letting Go of Envy and Jealousy
Volume 115: Fear of Spiders, Arachnophobia
Volume 116: Fear of Dogs or Cats
Volume 117: Fear of Strangers, Xenophobia
Volume 118: Excessive Worries, Generalized Anxiety
Volume 119: Strengthening Sense of Responsibility
Volume 120: Unrequited Love, Heartache
Volume 121: Work-Life Balance
Volume 122: Letting Go of Unattainable Goals
Volume 123: Allowing and Accepting Help
Volume 124: Letting Go of Adult Children
Volume 125: Tourette Syndrome
Volume 126: Life Changes and New Starts

Volume 127: Accepting Life in a Wheelchair
Volume 128: Understanding and Overcoming Homesickness
Volume 129: Understanding and Overcoming Wanderlust
Volume 130: Dizziness, Meniere's Disease
Volume 131: Overcoming Aggression
Volume 132: Cutting and Self-Harm
Volume 133: Hair Pulling, Trichotillomania
Volume 134: Postpartum Depression
Volume 135: For Relatives of Dementia Patients
Volume 136: Self-Harm, Artificial Disorders
Volume 137: Activating Self-Healing Powers
Volume 138: Preventing Depression Relapse
Volume 139: Reactive Psychoses, Follow-Up
Volume 140: Obsessive Thoughts and Impulses
Volume 141: Compulsive Checking
Volume 142: Compulsive Counting, Symmetry Obsession
Volume 143: Compulsive Washing, Cleanliness Obsession
Volume 144: Compulsive Questioning
Volume 145: Dissociative Paralysis
Volume 146: Phantom Pain
Volume 147: Overcoming Complaining
Volume 148: Hay Fever, Pollen Allergy
Volume 149: Sexual Abuse, Victim Support
Volume 150: Standing Strong Against Sexism, #metoo
Volume 151: Binge Eating
Volume 152: Overcoming Thoughts of Revenge
Volume 153: Detachment from the Aggressor, Stockholm Syndrome
Volume 154: Courage to Separate
Volume 155: Chronic Fatigue, Exhaustion
Volume 156: Fear of the Future, Existential Anxiety
Volume 157: Excessive Worry About Children
Volume 158: Fear of Failure

Volume 159: Ending Distrust and Control
Volume 160: Dejection, Dysphoria
Volume 161: Boreout, Chronic Boredom
Volume 162: Bipolar Disorders, Relapse Prevention
Volume 163: Mania, Relapse Prevention
Volume 164: Nihilism, Feelings of Worthlessness
Volume 165: Thumb Sucking
Volume 166: Being Brave
Volume 167: Being Proud
Volume 168: Overcoming Shyness
Volume 169: Being Able to Delegate Responsibility
Volume 170: Being Able to Show Emotions
Volume 171: Letting Go of Guilt, Victim Support
Volume 172: Processing Guilt, Offender Support
Volume 173: Mood Swings, Cyclothymia
Volume 174: Lack of Drive, Vital Sadness
Volume 175: Hearing Voices with Reality Reference
Volume 176: Confident Communication
Volume 177: Standing Up for Oneself
Volume 178: Taking New Paths
Volume 179: Confident Job Application
Volume 180: No Longer Being Taken Advantage Of
Volume 181: End of Submissiveness
Volume 182: Depressive Numbness
Volume 183: Mood Drops, Affective Incontinence
Volume 184: Mood Instability
Volume 185: Somatoform Disorders
Volume 186: Stomach Ulcer, Psychosomatic
Volume 187: Accepting Amputation
Volume 188: Overcoming and Letting Go of Hatred
Volume 189: Ending Accusations
Volume 190: Allowing Tears, Being Able to Cry

Volume 191: Finding and Sorting Repressed Feelings
Volume 192: Somatoform Pain
Volume 193: Living Autonomously
Volume 194: Anhedonia, Joylessness
Volume 195: Persistent Sadness
Volume 196: Obesity, Food Addiction
Volume 197: Parents of Abused Children
Volume 198: Letting Go and Letting Be
Volume 199: Childhood Sexual Abuse
Volume 200: Fear of Loss

www.ingramcontent.com/pod-product-compliance
Lightning Source LLC
Chambersburg PA
CBHW030501220526
45464CB00006B/2601